KRIYA

THE SCIENCE OF SELF-REALIZATION

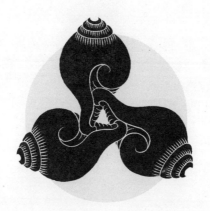

KRIYA YOGA

THE SCIENCE OF SELF REALIZATION

KRIYA YOGA
THE SCIENCE OF SELF-REALIZATION

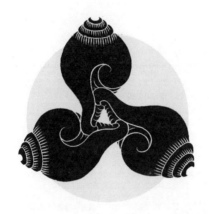

J.R. SANTIAGO

BOOK FAITH INDIA
Delhi

KRIYA YOGA : THE SCEINCE OF SELF-REALIZATION

Published by
BOOK FAITH INDIA
414-416 Express Tower
Azadpur Commercial Complex
Delhi, India 110033
Tel. [91-11] 713-2459. Fax [91-11] 724-9674
E-mail: pilgrim@del2.vsnl.net.in

Distributed by
PILGRIMS BOOK HOUSE
P.O.Box 3872
Kathmandu, Nepal
Tel. [977-1] 424942. Fax [977-1] 424943.
E-mail: pilgrims@wlink.com.np
WebSite: pilgrimsbooks.com

Varanasi Branch
PILGRIMS BOOK HOUSE
B 27/98-A-8, Durga Kund
Varanasi, India 221001
Tel. [91-542] 314060. Fax [91-542] 314059, 312788
E-mail: pilgrim@lw1.vsnl.net.in

Artwork by Dr. Sasya
Layout by Naresh Subba

1st Edition
Copyright © 1999 Book Faith India

ISBN 81-7303-184-3

Printed in India

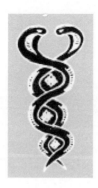

The aim of Yoga is Self-realization

"Self-realization is the knowing – in body, mind and soul — that we are one with the Omnipresence of God; that we do not pray that He comes to us, that we are not merely near Him at all times, but that God's ominipresence is our omnipresence; that we are just as much a part of Him now as we ever will be. All we have to do is improve our knowing."

— Sri Sri Paramahansa Yogananda

CONTENTS

Foreword   ix

Introduction   x

1.   Yoga : Definition   1

2.   Yoga : The Science of Enlightenment   7

3.   Patanjali's Yoga   19

4.   Kriya Yoga : History   33

5.   Kriya Yoga : Discipline & Techniques   43

6.   Kriya Yoga Meditation   49

Bibliography   64

Foreword

Yoga, the science of enlightenment, has become popular all over the world. Nearly everyone appears to know yoga. Nothing has spread so quickly in the last half century as yoga.

This interest must have been initially inspired by the publication of the *Autobiography of a Yogi* by Paramahansa Yogananda both in India and the United States. It is the story of a young boy who was inspired to become a renunciant, to follow the spiritual path. Eventually being initiated into Kriya Yoga discipline, he went to the United States where he gave a lecture and introduced Kriya Yoga.

Yoga is not a religion; it is really more a science, but the essence of religion is intrinsic in the discipline. It is timeless and its appeal is universal. One can remain faithful to his religion and still practice yoga.

It sprang up immediately after the Second World War with generally the young generation picking it up and spreading it all over the world. The Hippie Generation had sought to transform the world with the basic principle of 'Make Love Not War'. They evinced simultaneously both hope and despair. The latter brought about the introduction of psychotropic drugs. The world economy was getting better but there were problems that assailed the young.

It is an irony of life that economically developed countries, the prosperous western countries, produced social problems particularly for the young people. The young, inspired by Paramahansa Yogananda's book, flocked to the subcontinent and as a consequence this led to the Indian swamis going to the West to teach Hindu philosophy and yoga followed in their wake by Buddhist lamas.

Eastern philosophy taught that human beings have an inherent divine heritage, and that human suffering could be alleviated. It recommends yoga as a panacea for human ailments and problems.

This brief work on Kriya Yoga introduces one of the best yoga disciplines extant today. Efforts have been made to make it comprehensive, and because it is one of the best, some aspects of its processes are kept secret, simply to prevent it from suffering any modifications. For those who are interested in pursuing a deeper study of Kriya Yoga they can always communicate with the Self-Realization Fellowship in Los Angeles, California, or with the Yogoda Satsanga Society of India in Bihar, India.

Introduction

This introductory work is mainly based on *Patanjali's Yoga Sutras*, a broad treatise on yoga. Kriya yoga is a complex of techniques apparently culled from other disciplines, mostly from the Kundalini Yoga of Swami Shivananda. It requires strict and rigid discipline, adherence to rules and regulations, and therefore is not easy.

There appears to be four stages and each one has to be passed fully and completely, before moving on to the next stage. It is complex and difficult, requiring dedication and determination to succeed. It is considered the fastest method for achieving results. The essential requirement is to have patience and perseverance until the goal is attained.

The study course is traditional and includes doctrines, scriptures, mind and consciousness, the physical organs and the psychic energy centers in the human body. There are mystical ramifications inherent in its practice. It is said to liberate consciousness.

Depending on karmic disposition of a disciple he can attain the goal within a few months. This brief overview on Kriya Yoga is intended for those who wish to test its validity. Faith is strengthened in the testing. And faith must not be 'blind', but must be based on knowledge, that is, knowledge that is experienced. It is then faith that becomes unassailable.

This is an altogether different area of study. It is esoteric and thus concepts are not entirely easy to grasp. They are in Sanskrit and terms used have very broad meaning.

Spiritual concepts and their definitions are often vague. This volume simplifies them for easier understanding.

Authors on Kriya Yoga refuse to explain fully the meditation techniques and procedures in their books. They want the purity of the traditional transmission to be preserved by the yogic tradition of oral instruction.

They have strong reason to do so, because very often the text, with its esoteric vocabulary and manner of expressing spiritual ideas, could be ambiguous and might lead to confusion.

For this reason, spiritual enlightenment by oral instruction is preferred. A guru, is then able to answer the disciple's questions until vague concepts have been clearly learned.

This short work presents a broad overview of Kriya Yoga. It is one of the few works that presents this secret, mystical practice in public forum.

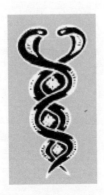

1

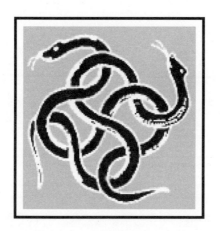

YOGA : DEFINITION

Yoga : Definition

Yoga is a philosophy and a science. The philosophy is the doctrine of the 'Divine Within', which claims that humanity has a divine heritage. And the science is the method of meditation that verifies and confirms the doctrine. In yoga the philosophy and science are intrinsic, inseparable, and reinforce each other.

Yoga is the science of the control or mastery of the mind.

In its broad ordinary usage the term 'yoga' means 'union' or 'integration'. The English word 'to yoke' derives its etymological origin from this Sanskrit word. In a specific context it has come to mean 'spiritual union' with the Absolute, which brings about a mystical event – self-realization – which in turn leads to enlightenment, and from enlightenment to final liberation. This is defined as freedom achieved through perfect yoga.

The term in its broad and common usage has become synonymous with 'method', and method means 'work' which in Sanskrit translates into the term 'kriya', the root word of which is based on the word 'karma' which means 'to do' or 'to act'. Thus 'kriya' also means 'work or action or ritual. Any work or action or ritual is called 'kriya'. And any method in yoga, ordinary or specialized is called 'kriya yoga' which means 'work toward yoga'. It must be noted however that a distinct system called 'kriya yoga' has evolved with its own specific and special techniques and processes entirely different from other yoga disciplines.

Patanjali's definition of yoga is 'the effort to separate Reality from the non-Real' and also 'to calm the mind'. This is not surprising. Sanskrit words very often have almost infinite ramifications and therefore numerous meanings, but each reinforcing or related to each other to sustain the motif or significance of a single concept. He also defined it as 'the neutralization of the alternating waves in consciousness; it is the cessation of the modifications of the mind-stuff. The main purpose is the removal of suffering and attainment of timeless bliss.'

Here therefore are quite a few distinct definitions, which apparently are not actually contradictory but complement each other. On one hand yoga is a struggle for union or integration, on the other hand it is an 'effort to separate Reality' or 'to calm the mind'. Yoga is union with Reality, but actually Reality is the spirit or *paramatman*, which is inherently a natural integral part of a human body. It is already in union with the body as claimed in the Tantric doctrine of the 'Divine Within', but it still requires effort to know and recognize it from other parts or essence of the human body. And it requires calming the mind to see it.

The disciple must learn to distinguish Reality from the non-Real and must recognize it when it finally appears to him. When Reality is seen in deep meditation he is said to have realized his own nature. The experience in deep meditation is ineffable, enveloped in a kind of nirvana, when Reality appears. This is called 'cosmic consciousness' and regarded as true knowledge because it has been experienced. The elan vital or divine spark is a round brilliant dazzling burnished gold in color. It is not spherical.

Patanjali's purpose is first to know how to separate the Real from the non-Real, for even if the initiate had already experienced union, if he had no knowledge of the divine spark he would not have any ideas he had already realized the goal of yoga. This is the reason as shall be seen later why he set the preliminary stages essential to meditation.

It is only when it holds you in its embrace that the Real reveals itself. It occurs when the initiate's mind becomes calm and placid, in fact when everything is obliterated, the phenomenal world, body sensation, and the flow of mind ceases and there is only a profound Silence which envelopes the initiate. It is therefore 'kriya' or 'work' to realize the philosophy. The end result is mystical. It is for this reason that yoga is defined as a mystic science.

This mystical experience, however, must be taken on faith. It is to attempt to experiment with the scientific method of yogic meditation, to determine whether or not it will bring or effect the result being pursued. If the meditation is successful it will verify and method and confirm the philosophy on which it is based.

4

It is an individual undertaking, no one can help him, he alone must attempt it. And when he experiences the same result that had been revealed to him by his guru he confirms the philosophy and verifies the authenticity of the method. It is experiential, and the knowledge acquired is by direct vision. It is supersensory. This experience reinforces and confirms knowledge already known.

Yoga, along with other spiritual practices, evolved out of man's attempt to resolve his problems, but it was discovered that the fundamental problem is his alienation from his divine heritage. The 'Divine Within' doctrine emphasizes that the human body is in fact the 'Temple of the Divine'. Yoga therefore became fundamental path to salvation: it provides the 'kriya' to seek and unite with the Absolute.

To seek the eternal is not easy. Yogic meditation is not easy. It is extremely difficult, but not impossible. Nothing is easy, but nothing in yoga is impossible. In fact the benefits acquired through yoga are said to be immense, even beyond reckoning. Nothing is certain; the teachings of the masters have to be taken on faith. It provides the possibility of having an adventure in another dimension.

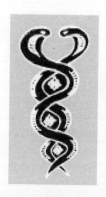

2

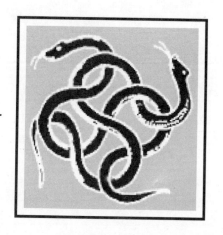

YOGA
THE SCIENCE OF ENLIGHTENMENT

Yoga : The Science Of Enlightenment

Yoga is considered as India's unique and deathless contribution to the world's treasury of human knowledge. In Sanskrit the term yoga means 'union'. It has the same connotation as the English word 'to yoke', which also means to 'harness' power or energy for a certain purpose.

In the spiritual context it evolved into a secret mystical practice which has been kept within a special group of people, not freely revealed to the uninitiated. Traditionally it was taught only to a chosen few, and inevitably it was eventually forgotten.

It was fundamentally a religious principle with meditation as its method, a form of inner worship with the ultimate goal of attaining union with the Eternal. It is experimental and experiential and therefore an individual and personal form of inner worship: the experiment is done in meditation, which puts the worshipper into the Silent Realm in union with the Almighty. The process involves getting deeper into the Silent Realm until the worshipper gets into the state of *samadhi.*

The prehistoric tribal folk cult form of worship involved offering sacrifices and the most common was the fire ritual. Prior to this form of worship the tribal folk religion was called *sanatan,* the worship of nature, of the rocks, the trees, caves and rivers, which brought about the building of primitive shrines in every nook and corner of the land.

In the tribal agrarian community the Goddess of fertility emerged, but the worship of nature was not discarded, continued, and is still practiced to these days. It never apparently suffered any permutation in its evolution; it has remained unchanged. Thus it is only in the subcontinent where prehistoric form of worship can be traced and observed, but whose origin is lost in the mist of time.

There must have been some social changes most particularly when urban areas, due to economic prosperity, began to develop, which brought about the transformation of society. In the vast rural regions of India the form of worship, as has been noted, never suffered any changes, and thus it could only have been in the urban areas where another form of worship must have evolved.

This development marks a watershed in the Indian cultural and religious evolution. This new form of worship is known as yoga. It is very old: there is only archaeological evidence of its existence and practice dug up in the Indus Valley Civilization, circa 3000 BC, which is also known as the Harappan Civilization.

The archaeological artifacts dug up in Moenjodaro include steatite seals, one of which displays a man, presumably Shiva as the Lord of Nature, the 'dark god of a dark people', known then by the epithet Balaji, surrounded by animals. Another shows him in the yogic posture of absorption or *samadhi*. Shiva in fact is said to have revealed Tantra and the practice of yogic meditation to mankind. He is regarded as the 'Patron of Yogies'.

In the *Bhagavad Gita,* however, Krishna claims, , to have introduced yoga to an ancient illuminato, Vivasrat, who gave it to Manu, the great legislator, who in turn instructed Ikshwaku on yoga. Yoga was passed on from generation to generation until through the indifference and neglect of the ecclesiastics was forgotten and was lost. In the time of the *Mahabaratta* he was to reintroduce it to Arjuna.

In reference to the Mahabaratta during Krishna's lifetime, the Saraswati River that flowed westward, drained by the Sea of Arabia, was still in existence for Krishna was to sail down the river all the way down to Dhwarka. It was the Mahabaratta in fact which inspired a prominent Indian archaeologist to request NASA to take satellite photographs of the region traversed by the river: this is now made up of Rajasthan, Maharastra and Gujarat. The NASA photographs of the region showed vestiges of the river's route westward.

This means that the Mahabaratta antedates the existence of the Harappan Civilization. And when the river dried up preceded by the desertification of Mongolia and Central Asia the Old Aryan tribes settled on the banks of the Saraswati moved out, with some of them settling on the banks of the Indus River.

The Old Aryans called themselves 'wanderers' or 'nomads'. The second batch of Aryan tribes that arrived in 1700 BC, two centuries after the Harappan Civilization had been devastated by flood, called themselves 'nobles'. They brought with them a pottery inferior to the sophistication of the remnants of the Harappan culture. But they understood the language of the Old Aryans they found settled on the banks of the Indus.

It must be during this period, the Vedic Age, that the Vedas (truth) were written. They were made up of the religious and philosophical discourses, which were passed on from generation to generation by oral tradition. They made up the religious heritage of the indigenous people, which were subsequently taken up by the Old Aryans. There is a great reason to support this assertion for everything in the Vedas came from Tantra, the tribal folk way of life and way of knowledge.

Yoga is Tantric, and it appears not to have been noted previously, but appeared in the *Mahabaratta* epic. There were, however, treatises on yoga, which eventually were collected by Patanjali. Patanjali's period is fairly vague: authors could not agree on a definite and specific period. Some authors claim the Yoga Sutras were written in the 4th century BC, while others claimed a much later date, 4th century AD, while still others suggested they may have been written 'one thousand years ago', which means the 10th century AD.

What one could deduce from Patanjali's Yoga Sutra was that the practice of yogic meditation and its requirements, was already fully developed. And apparently it has retained its original form and purity. This is the yoga that is now spreading all over the world.

Tantrism may have been originally concerned with the study of human nature and the physical form, which led to the discovery of psychic energy centers, the chakras, located in the spinal column, along with the kundalini, the Serpent Power, called Shakti. And the doctrine of the 'Divine Within' evolved. The experience of *participation mystique* confirmed the doctrine. This was the reason the Vedics could not compete with the Tantrics and failed in their effort to subvert Tantrism.

This may have begun with the science of mantra, the repetition of sounds along with pranayama, the control of the process of breathing. These were perhaps the early methods in yogic meditation. There are other methods, which include the asanas or physical exercises with postures (mudras) and the sexo-yogic method or coitus, a sublimated form of connubium. Yoga is actually a union of the male and female principles.

Central to the science of yoga is the awakening of the occult cerebrospinal centers, the chakras, known as astral lotuses. These are unseen, not visible even to the modern most powerful microscopes; they are still not located by scientists and doctors, who study in detail human anatomy, its organs and the nervous system.

This is of course mystifying: the fact that they have been discovered and known by the ancient sages of India raises a question that is almost impossible to answer. This, however, also reveals the power of yoga, that it can enable man to know by direct vision aspects of the human body that are ordinarily not visible and known. Yoga was the most powerful system available to the rishis of India.

It is really quite astonishing how they came to discover these secret aspects in the human body. There are seven of these chakras, all located along the spinal column from the base up to the head where the seventh chakra is located. Besides these psychic centers they discovered also kundalini, so called because it is coiled at the base of the spine. This is the real power that provides energy to the human body. It is also known as the Serpent Power: this is the goddess Shakti.

Shakti has to be aroused to move up to the different psychic centers until it reaches the seventh chakra, known as the sahasrara chakra. And when Shakti, the feminine principle, reaches the seventh chakra, it unites with the resident deity, Shiva, the male principle. The result is yoga. Another incredible discovery is the presence of the divine spark in the heart. Many more will be revealed in this brief overview on yoga. They are on the whole mentioned in the Yoga Sutras of Patanjali, which by deduction could be regarded as really an incredibly profound system of power.

On the superficial level yoga meditation appears simple and easy, but on a deeper level, thinking about it, it becomes extremely difficult. Progress is step by step, and it will take years before any positive result could be observed.

How easy or difficult it is apparently depends on the karma of the individual aspirant. For some success may come easily within a few weeks or months, but for others it may take years or even many lifetimes before the ultimate goal can be achieved. This inequality among human beings is mainly due to karma, the law of cause and effect, the principle of equilibrium. It is karma that creates individuality, which makes people different from one another.

The success of an initiate therefore depends on his karma, which determines the possibility of his having a successful yoga. If he has good *samskara* or good tendencies success will be fairly easy. Samskara determines human character, which could have good or bad propensities. But whatever its present nature or character it can be transformed. This nevertheless requires great effort. The purpose is to be able to remain calm and one-pointed: this is essential for a successful yogic meditation.

Yoga requires learning the process and the requirements of meditation. The first essential step is concentration, for by this method thought-waves or even emotions have to be controlled. To achieve concentration some practice with some objects or symbols, such as a single lighted candle or a bull's-eye target, or the portrait of a deity. It is usually recommended to the aspirant to concentrate either on the tip of his nose or the Third Eye known also as the 'spiritual eye' or the 'inner eye' or 'eye of intention' located at the point between the eyebrows. This is actually the sixth chakra regarded as a holy spot, the point of consciousness. The most common is concentrating on pranayama, the process of rhythmic breathing.

The purpose of concentration is to achieve one-pointedness, and this requires stopping the flow of thought-waves, also known as 'mental modifications'. This means all thought-waves regardless of whether they are good or bad. There must be complete cessation of the flow of mind with consciousness channeled towards self-knowledge. Non-attachment is involved here. It is not analogous to indifference, but is actually the essence of discrimination, to distinguish Reality from the non-real. As has been noted the aspirant need not consider whether a thought is good or bad, but he must exercise non-attachment or discrimination, and concentrate mainly on achieving one-pointedness for a successful yoga.

The man who achieves perfect yoga is described as being 'liberated'. However, this does not mean the immediate cessation of the practice. He must continue with his meditation until he is firmly established in super-consciousness. The words, thoughts and actions of a liberated man are said to be like 'burnt seeds', no longer linked to karma. The remainder of his earthly life will be governed by karmas already in existence before his liberation.

For success in meditation faith, energy and dedication are essential. One must have faith, and to have faith is to give the practice a try, and to give it a try one must have energy, and to have energy one must have dedication or determination to succeed. The initiate must keep himself absorb in meditation until he finally attains success. Devotion to a deity is also recommended, and so is the chanting of OM mantra, and pranayama, particularly the practice of expelling or retaining breath. Prana is a universal energy, which is conscious; it is a vital energy that comes with breath. To control the mind is a psychophysical problem and pranayama is a psychophysical method of calming the mind. Experiments and experience have actually proved that deep steady inhalation and exhalation calm the mind.

And so does the chanting of the mantra. Both pranayama and chanting of mantra are psychophysical methods to a spiritual end. Both methods are also employed in awakening latent psychic powers in the human body. Both are very powerful means of making the mind one-pointed. When concentration becomes fixed and established the breath or mantra could be focussed on certain psychic energy centers, or any sensitive part of the body, either to sharpen the sense organs or awaken latent powers to release energy required.

Both methods are actually physically energizing: breathing exercises and chanting mantra are not merely relaxing but energize the body by filling it with prana. When their effects are experienced in experiments they provide encouragement to continue the practice. It is therefore not only for spiritual purpose but for physical well-being, and as a consequence produces a balanced frame of mind.

In the *Bhagavad Gita,* Krishna described the practice as 'offering the inhaling breath into the exhaling breath, and offering the exhaling breath into the inhaling breath, the yogi neutralizes both breath; thus, he releases prana from the heart and brings life-force under his control.' It is to fix the focus on the spiritual eye and control the senses and consciousness, and to banish desire, fear and anger.

The ancient yogis discovered that the secret of cosmic consciousness is intimately linked with breath-mastery. This is a simple method in which human blood is decabornized and recharged with oxygen, the atoms of which are transmuted into life current to rejuvenate the brain and the spinal centers: this prevents the decay of tissues. The body decay is arrested by an additional supply of prana by cooling the action of the heart and the lungs.

All this, nevertheless, requires the simultaneous development of virtue, such as friendliness or compassion towards all sentient beings, and being indifferent towards the wicked and avoiding 'resisting evil' with evil.

When concentration has finally been achieved to a higher degree it could be focussed on the inner light residing in the heart. The yogis of ancient times called this 'the Lotus of the Heart', because they have seen it in the form of a lotus. They emphasized the importance of focusing on this inner light in meditation. The Kaivalta Upanishad advises the aspirant 'to enter the lotus of the heart' and mediate there.

This does not mean physical entry as this is impossible: this means bringing consciousness into the heart and meditate on the inner light. The Chandogya Upanishad states that:

"Within the heart... there is a chamber which has the shape of a lotus, and within it dwells that which is sought after, inquired about and realized."

"Within it are heaven and earth, the sun, the moon, the lightning and all the stars. Whatever is in the macrocosm is in the microcosm also."

The Mundaka Upanishad says:

"Within the lotus of the heart He dwells, where the nerves of the heart meet like the spokes of a wheel. Meditate upon Him as OM, and you may easily cross the ocean of darkness. In the effulgent lotus of the heart dwells Brahman, passionless and indivisible. He is pure. He is the light of all lights. The knower of Brahman attains Him."

Concentration can also be fixed on a divine being, or a sacred dream, or any divine form, which appeals to the aspirant.

According to Vedanta, the philosophy based on the Vedas, the Atman in the human body is covered by three layers of sheaths. The outermost is the physical sheath, the layer for gross matter; and below this is the subtle sheath composed of the inner essence of things: this is the stuff of the spirit world. The third is the causal sheath: it contains the ego sense, which makes the individual see himself and the phenomenal universe as separate entities.

These three sheaths cover and separate the Atman. Actually the problem is basically ignorance, which can be removed by knowledge. Knowledge must come first, before discrimination could distinguish what is

Real from the non-real. Knowledge and discrimination cleanse the sheaths. And union with the Atman is attained in deep meditation through the power of one-pointed concentration.

When one has achieved the power of undivided concentration — one-pointedness — he is said to have become a yogi. One therefore can become a yogi when he has achieved control over his body and mind. When the mind is finally controlled and comes into union with the object of concentration it attains oneness or identification with it. This is known as *samadhi*, the state of yoga. Samadhi is a blissful super-conscious state in which a yogi perceives the identity of the individual and the cosmic spirit. It is described as ultra-sensual bliss experienced in super-consciousness, and is considered far superior to sense delights.

There are three different levels of samadhi. No kind of samadhi is attainable until the mind has been controlled to allow consciousness to acquire the tremendous power of concentration. The lowest kind of samadhi is known as Savitarka Samadhi: this refers to 'awareness'. It is usual in this form of samadhi for the initiate to focus on a gross object, usually an aid to concentration, and when union, for instance, is achieved with a lighted candle the initiate is still aware of the candle as a candle. This means that identification with the object of concentration is incomplete.

This is also known as Sabikalpa Samadhi: the initiate experiences the initial contact with God. The initiate's consciousness merges with the cosmic spirit; his life force is withdrawn from the body, which appears dead or motionless and rigid, but he is aware of his physical condition of suspended animation.

Next is the Nirvitarka Samadhi, which translates 'without deliberation'. It is a higher stage of samadhi, a deeper form, which means the initiate has merged or identified with the object of concentration and has lost his awareness or consciousness of it. The initiate has finally been able to control thought-waves or his reactions to the object of concentration, and to know nothing of it, except 'the thing-in-itself'. This is known as transcendental knowledge. This samadhi is also otherwise known as Nirvikalpa Samadhi.

There are also two kinds of samadhi when concentration is on subtle objects: the Savichara Samadhi is yoga with awareness still with the initiate; and Nirvichara Samadhi is without any awareness of the object of concentration.

These four kinds of samadhi are regarded to be with 'seeds' of desire, which are considered dangerous to the practice of yoga meditation. This is the main reason the aspirant for the yogic experience is advised to practice non-attachment.

When samadhi is experienced it encourages the yogi to cultivate non-attachment and continue to work for the higher stages. When one has attained Nirvichara samadhi the yogi's mind is said to become pure, and what knowledge he has acquired is said to be 'filled with truth'. The knowledge gained through samadhi is of a much higher order than knowledge acquired by inference and the scriptures, which is attained through the senses, which is regarded as ordinary, but what is acquired in samadhi is considered extraordinary.

This type of knowledge is considered supersensory, capable of confirming the truth of yoga teachings through direct experience in samadhi. To be a yogi one has to verify and confirm yoga teachings, and only through the practice of meditation can he attain supersensory knowledge. Swami Vivekananda was to say that:

"Realization is real religion... Religion is a severely practical and empirical kind of research. You take nothing on trust. You accept nothing but your experience. You move forward alone, step by step, like an explorer... to see what you will find. All that Patanjali or anybody else can do for you is to urge you to attempt the exploration and to offer certain hints and warnings which may be of help to you on your way."

The mind in Nirvichara Samadhi experiences direct supersensory knowledge, and this knowledge is 'filled with truth'. Whatever object you focus on is transformed by a power, which reveals the true 'thing-in-itself'. It presents you the real thing and this is transcendental knowledge. This is what is called 'grace'. It descends during samadhi. This knowledge is unknowable by the senses; it is thus considered a 'revelation'. And this brings a transformation of character for in the unitive state of samadhi a man becomes a saint.

His character is transformed because samadhi wipes out all the past impressions, and when the final impression made during samadhi dissolves then he enters into the highest kind of samadhi which is 'seedless' and this is called Nirivikalpa Samadhi. It is said to be 'seedless' because it no longer contains phenomenal impressions, no desire or attachment, but only pure and undifferentiated consciousness, and this is Brahman or the Godhead.

Sankaracharya, the greatest philosopher of India, described Nirvikalpa Samadhi as follows:

"There is a continuous consciousness of the unity of Atman and Brahman... All sense duality is obliterated... The man who is well established in this consciousness is said to be illumined.

"A man is said to be free even in this life when he is established in illumination. His bliss is unending. He almost forgets this world of awareness.

"Even though his mind is dissolved in Brahman, he is fully aware, free from ignorance of waking life. He is fully conscious but free from any craving. Such a man is said to be free in this life.

"For him the sorrows of this life are over. Though he possesses a finite body, he remains united with the Infinite. His heart knows no anxiety. Such a man is said to be free even in this life."

Reality is Brahman or Godhead. This does not mean that everything is illusion, for everything is Brahman. And for this reason the Godhead is fundamental and omnipresent. This concept of Reality expands man's perception; he sees deeper; the perception of an illumined saint ranges over the whole scale, from the gross to the subtle, and from the subtle to the Absolute.

And it is only he who knows the nature of this universe.

Dr. C.G. Jung, the famous Swiss psychologist, wrote, "...by reason of its breadth and depth, its venerable age, its doctrine and method, which include every phase of life, it promises ...possibilities... It combines the bodily and spiritual with each other in an extraordinarily complete way... This unity creates a psychological disposition which makes possible intuition that transcends consciousness."

Yoga leads to a conscious direction of one's mind and life. It is a science, which has a universal appeal. In the *Bhagavad Gita* Krishna was to instruct Arjuna thus: "The yogi is greater than the body-disciplining ascetics, greater even than the followers of the path of wisdom or the path of action; be thou, O disciple Arjuna, a yogi."

This system leads to Kaivalya (Absoluteness), the realization of Reality – the Truth.

3

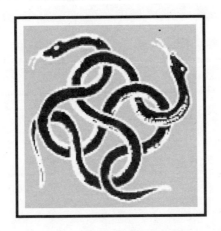

PATANJALI'S YOGA

PATANJALI'S YOGA

Patanjali's yoga sutras preserved the esoteric knowledge of the mystical system for posterity. It makes up the basics of all the yoga methods that later developed, which followed the fundamental principles, but diverged from each other as the different gurus or schools of thought evolved their own special and particular techniques.

It can safely be deduced that even earlier in his time, the original Tantric yoga revealed by Shiva or introduced and taught by Krishna, had already undergone great changes for there were not only a single treatise on yoga but many which Patanjali collated and turned into a single work.

Although perhaps the different treatises on yoga may have had diverging techniques the teachings or prescribed requirements must have been the same for them all: it was basically kriya (work) towards yoga. The different techniques, although not similar, work toward the same goal. Some or all of these techniques must have been combined and developed into one particular system by the different masters: it was inspired by the desire to make improvements on methods, which they taught their disciples.

As a consequence many methods with different special systems emerged. It is not very clear, mainly due to its broad scope, if Patanjali had described his yoga method as Raja Yoga — Royal Yoga. The translators and commentators of his yoga sutras described his method as Royal Yoga. This is the best among the four major systems, apparently because it combines the three other methods: the Bhakti Yoga or devotional yoga, Jnana Yoga, the way through knowledge, and Karma Yoga, the way through work.

There are other methods with varying physical techniques, such as the Hatha Yoga, the way to make the body perfect, and the use of mantra and pranayama. These different methods are mentioned in the yoga sutras; but they appear apart from each other, not combined for a single method. Only the Raja Yoga appears to combine all the other three major methods.

The Royal Yoga is eight-limbed: the first five limbs cover the processes to attain yoga; the last three limbs pertain to the acquisition of 'siddhis' or supernatural power: this may be perhaps the reason the Royal Yoga is viewed as the best. Although Patanjali did not specifically describe his yoga the sutras actually defined it as such. It is not easy but extremely difficult. It involves the total transformation of character, and even the personality of the aspirant. He has to go against his own human nature, even to the extent of renouncing mundane life: it is mainly to become a yogi or to acquire 'siddhis' and become a 'Siddha Yogi'.

The Royal Yoga is the highest type and thus it is the best, but also the most difficult, for it does not involve one method but several techniques, and as shall be noted all laws or principles governing human life. It is therefore holistic in its approach: it is a whole and complete view of human life. It is also thus severely rigid as a monk's life: it is not seeking material comfort but God. One cannot be pragmatic and desultory in this method.

What follows is a brief summary of *Patanjali's Yoga Sutras*, but it presents a fairly comprehensive concept of the whole system. It is a brief exegesis of the complex method to give an idea of what is involved.

Since the Kriya Yoga of Babaji is primarily based on Patanjali's sutras this short overview will later be expanded as supplements will be included in explaining Babaji's yoga system. It is not really different therefore from the Royal Yoga, but becomes distinct and distinguishable in its use of different techniques of the different principal methods.

The aspirant who wishes to follow the spiritual path to become a yogi must work toward yoga: this is actually *kriya yoga*. He must practice austerity, study the scriptures, and dedicate all the fruits of his labor to God. In practicing austerity he must exercise temperance, moderateness in everything, in body, mind and speech — in actions, thoughts and words. Austerity of the body means reverence for deities, the sages and teachers; the practice of harmlessness, frankness or honesty and sincerity, also physical cleanliness, mental and sexual purity. Austerity of the mind includes mental evenness or calmness, compassion for others, withdrawal of the mind from sense objects. It also means integrity in meditation upon the Atman — the divine spark — in the heart. Austerity of speech is the practice of not causing pain or harm by bearing false witness against others: it is always to remain truthful.

This is actually the practice of self-control, the control of the senses, and this requires knowledge and discrimination. Knowledge is required to be able to practice discrimination. Hence, the study of the scriptures and the need for a guru. He who controls the mind (the senses are linked to the mind) reaches the end of the journey and arrives at his goal.

The initiate must perform ritual worship, for worship is not simply a display of devotion, but worship is also an aid to concentration. And this is mainly because rituals are very elaborate, and performance requires unbroken attention. The worshipper must focus his attention — his consciousness — on each successive step or act to recall the thought or aim behind each act. He becomes too busy to think of anything else. Thus in ritual worship thought and action form a continuous chain, and this is particularly true in the mandala-worship.

A man interested in attaining self-realization must start from the very beginning: in the ordinary worship involving elementary or preliminary steps towards a higher form, such as meditation. This is because man usually begins worshipping for physical security, for material things he needs in life. But in meditation he now seeks spiritual security; he is seeking the Absolute, to attain union with It.

The requirement to study involves the reading of sacred scriptures and other holy books, and studying their meaning and significance. This also includes doing japa, the chanting of mantra repeatedly with the use of japa-beads. The effect of mantra must also be studied along with the use of a rosary. This is actually an aid in retaining and conserving energy and also in concentration. It keeps the mind focused on the beads and on chanting of the mantra; it is to remove unnecessary thought-waves and emotions thus conserving energy besides becoming one-pointed and attaining deeper concentration. This technique keeps the chaotic world away, at bay so to say, when the initiate focuses on the Absolute during the chanting of the mantra repeatedly on his japa-beads. It is a practical aid and method.

While cultivating or practicing virtue the initiate is also learning the essential steps in the procedure of yoga and acquiring the essential knowledge required. All three are done simultaneously altogether with the effect that each stage reinforces the others. There is a wholeness to the process: virtue is practiced, learning is undertaken, while at the same time exercising the different methods of focussing attention to make it one-pointed. This is the most important aspect of the procedure, in which purity of mind and body is worked for with just this basic technique. Acquiring knowledge also sustains this technique.

The requirement to dedicate the fruits of his labor is considered of vital importance. This is known as karma yoga: it is a way toward yoga through the performance of spiritually dedicated labor or action to God. The whole life of a karma yogi becomes an unending worship: every act is done as an offering to God. Offering the fruits of labor to God is defined as non-attachment: that the devotee has done his best in his work is his only legitimate reward. The best, not the second best, has to be offered to God. There is thus a sense of fulfillment in the karma yogi even if his work in the world is a failure.

Success or failure to the karma yogi does not matter to him anymore, because he knows he is not the one working; it is God working through him. God experiences the whole work as He is also the doer. It is then God who fails or succeeds through the labor of the karma yogi. This is an exercise in absolute non-attachment towards the fruits of his labor.

In his study the man on a spiritual path learns the causes of human sufferings, and these are ignorance, egoism, attachment, and the desire to cling to life. These are the obstacles in the spiritual pursuit of concentration and enlightenment.

Ignorance is the fundamental problem: it is the cause of all other problems or causes of human sufferings. Because of ignorance, offence against the Atman, which is in our own true nature is committed. This is regarded as the ultimate 'sin', which is the alienation from the Reality within. This is an obstacle to enlightenment, and the penalty is contained within the self and is thus automatic as self identifies with the ego, which results in suffering. 'Sin' brings in alienation, caused by wrong identification which in turn is mainly due to ignorance, and 'sin' brings in retribution by causing sufferings. This is true with rajasic worldly people.

The Kena Upanishad defines the Atman thus:

> "At whose behest does the mind think? Who bids the body live? Who makes the tongue speak? Who is that effulgent Being that directs the eye to form and color, and the ear to sound? The Atman is the ear of the ear, the mind

of the mind, speech of the speech. He is also the breath of the breath, and eye of the eye. Having given up the false identification of the Atman with the senses and the mind, and knowing Atman to be Brahman, the wise becomes immortal."

The principle of non-attachment is neither indifference nor aversion. The spiritual aspirant must not love things of this world too much to be attached to them, but neither must he hate them, for aversion, like attachment, is a form of bondage. Hatred or aversion is just like attachment: to hate is to be linked up with the object hated. The aspirant therefore must develop dispassionate insight.

In this life apparently Nature has a purpose for humanity; for every individual: it is to make man journey towards total consciousness. Man thus is in the throes of evolution; he is still in the process of evolving towards perfection.

In this life man is subject to the law of karma, and other sub-principles governing his life, such as *samsara*, the cycle of birth and death. Whatever he does either speed or retard his progress towards full development. His life is continually conditioned by karma, and he either builds or removes his own obstacles to perfection or enlightenment. He is continually producing future karmas. Death does not end the process; it continues, for he is reborn with a new body, mind and character — the sum total of his karmic balance.

The doctrine of reincarnation is a concept that is undesirable, for it makes every individual directly responsible for his actions, thoughts and words – for his present condition in life.

The translators and commentators on Patanjali's yoga sutras say that most people do not like having responsibilities, even to themselves. And when they are reborn physically and economically underprivileged they blame the principle of heredity, circumstances and environment, or even blame God for everything, or even the political system, or the social atmosphere, or even the educational system. They have permanent excuse for all their weaknesses, failures and sufferings, and they curse fate.

The doctrine of reincarnation caused by karma is grim, but actually it implies a profound optimistic belief in justice and order in the universe. Thus no one escapes from his unjust acts, words or even thoughts, which are not only inimical to his fellowmen but also to himself.

Karma is a law involving cause and effect. For an unjust act the penalty may not come in a lifetime, but the next. It is inexorable in its effect, and for unjust acts he will also suffer the same unjust act, not necessarily from his previous victim but from other people. People therefore appear under mysterious prenatal curse, for they forget their own unjust acts when they are reborn, and it appears like a curse. According to Hinduism the individual himself can remove the curse, but he must realize his faults first, and then begin to act or behave responsibly towards others in his social milieu as well as toward himself.

Karma is what makes instincts and abilities, and this is the reason no identical twins are exactly the same. It is the cause of individual differentiation in humanity.

The Brihadaranyaka Upanishad has this to say about the fear of the experience of death:

"There are two states for man: the state in this world and the state in the next; there is also a third state, the state intermediate between these two, which can be likened to a dream. In the intermediate state a man experiences both the other states, that in this world and in the next; and the manner thereof is as follows:

"When he dies he lives only in the subtle body on which are left the impressions of his past deeds, and of these impressions he is aware, illumined as they are by the light of the Atman. The pure light of the Atman affords him light. Thus it is in the intermediate state he experiences the first state or that life in the world... And he foresees both the evils and blessings that will yet come to him, as these are determined by his conduct, good or bad, upon the earth, and by the character in which this conduct has resulted."

A man's karma determines his character on being reborn, and in his character exists latent tendencies. These tendencies when acted upon by thought or deeds will have consequences good or bad. Thus people resort to acts of merit in the belief these will produce pleasant results, but all experiences are considered 'painful', for even the pleasant experiences are a cause of bondage. The only true state of happiness is union with the Atman.

Past karmas can no longer be avoided; retribution is sure and relentless. But the present karma in this life can be avoided by dedicating the fruits of man's labor to God. The real problem is the false identification of the experience with the object of experience. Actually the one who experiences is the Atman, the real nature of a human being, for the Atman alone exists, 'one without a second'. It is only through Maya that the mystery of the present predicament of humanity can be perceived and deduced. The tragedy is identifying oneself with the object of experience. People thus are unaware of maya because of ignorance. And they remain in bondage as slaves of experience.

The Atman is everything; it is the essence of everything in the phenomenal universe.

Ignorance must be destroyed, and it can only be destroyed by knowledge gained by direct supersensory experience, not by ordinary senses. Direct supersensory experience can be obtained through yogic meditation in the attainment of samadhi. What is gained is the real or true knowledge. When by this means ignorance is destroyed man becomes free and independent.

Knowledge of the Atman is gained through seven stages:

1. The realization that the Atman is within the human body.
   As swami Vivekananda says, "it is the nearest of the near, is your own self, the reality of your life, body and soul."

2. The cessation of pain.
   The mind must turn inward to know the Atman. Knowledge destroys attachments and aversions, and frees man.

3. Attainment of Samadhi.
   This is attained in deep meditation resulting in union with the Atman, and this is self-realization and enlightenment.

4. The alteration of man's consciousness as a result of samadhi.
   The phenomenal universe is regarded only as a reflection of the Atman, like an image in a mirror. Now his actions are no longer motivated by selfish interests or attachment.

5. A realization dawns.
   After samadhi a man realizes that the mind and the objective world have both ended their service to the aspirant. They have already been used and transcended.

6. Impressions made by the gunas, these three principal elements of Nature fall away from the mind.

   The gunas are said to be again in a state of equilibrium. To understand the gunas these are three elements produced by the creation of the phenomenal universe.

7. When union with the Atman is attained.

   This is the final stage. The aspirant now becomes a yogi, never again to be deluded, peaceful and blessed with perfect knowledge.

The removal of impure impressions in the mind is the sole purpose of the spiritual discipline in the pursuit of yoga. The Atman is within and ever-present, and when the obstacles are removed the Atman is immediately revealed.

The eight limbs of Patanjali's yoga are rules and practices to be observed to clear the mind of its impurities.

They are as follow:

1. **Yama :** This is refraining from evil, such as harming others, and falsehood, theft, incontinence, and greed.

   Greed includes receiving gifts from the generosity of others with selfish interest.

   These are the basic rules of conduct, which must be practiced without any reservation at all times everywhere. There are no exceptions to the rule.

2. **Niyama :** These are observances in purity, contentment, mortification, study and devotion to God.

   Purity here means physical and mental purity. But usually these crop up on their own to teach man fearlessness, to develop non-fear of death.

3. **Asanas :** These involve physical exercises with postures. This is mainly Hatha Yoga for the perfection of the human body; but there are also exercises or mudras designed to awaken latent psychic forces in the body, such as the kundalini.

4. **Pranayama :** This is also physical: it is to control prana by a methodical rhythmic breathing system to increase pranic energy in the body and also to awaken latent psychic forces by chanting mantra.
5. **Pratyahara :** This is a psychophysical method of consciously withdrawing the mind from sense objects. It is to control the mind.
6. **Concentration (Dharana) :** This is the effort to make consciousness one-pointed for a successful yogic meditation.
7. **Meditation (Dhyana) :** This is now the process to attain self-realization.
8. **Absorption (Samadhi) :** This is the final stage: it occurs when aspirant attains self-realization and final liberation.

The successful practice of these eight limbs of yoga will effect changes in the mind, and therefore the character of the initiate will be transformed. Vivekananda was to say, "the first sign of your becoming religious is that you are becoming cheerful." Religious means here 'being tied to God.

Four Major Paths of Yoga:

1. **Bhakti Yoga :** This is the path of loving devotion to God. It is the cultivation of a direct and intense personal relationship with God by means of rituals, prayers and japa, the chanting of mantra. This is the simplest of all paths.
2. **Karma Yoga :** This is the path of God-dedicated actions. Bondage falls away, and the wheel of karma ceases to revolve. And God is known. This is the path best suited to energetic rajasic (dynamic) people.
3. **Jnana Yoga :** This is the path of intellectual discrimination, the analysis of the real nature of the phenomenal universe. The jnana yogi rejects all that is transient, apparent and superficial. He eliminates all these for the Real. It is not a path for ordinary people for it requires clarity of mind and tremendous intellectual power.

4. **Raja Yoga :** It is known as the Royal Yoga. Actually it is the yoga which combines all other paths. It is in the main concerned with the study of the body as a vehicle of spiritual energy: thus it studies psychic centers in the human body. It stresses the value of formal scientific meditation. It is suitable for monks or those of contemplative nature.

The Royal Yoga is so named because it is considered one of the best or the best of all methods. It combines in a complex system all the other three major paths, but it also involves in the discipline Hatha Yoga techniques, such as asanas and pranayama. Perhaps it takes only techniques of the asanas which are regarded as suitable to their system, such as the lotus posture with the feet drawn in and resting on the thighs. It makes one meditating sit still and erect.

The techniques involved in pranayama may have been taken as a whole for the Raja Yoga system. This is rhythmic breathing process, of stopping inhalation and exhalation. Breath can be stopped externally or internally or checked in mid-motion. It is regulated, and for its purpose time and place must be observed, and so are the fixed number of movement. Some stoppages could be brief and protracted. When the lungs have been emptied of air after exhalation the stoppage is described as external. If breath is checked after inhalation the stoppage is said to be internal. Breath could be stopped for a period of time. Central to pranayama technique is the control of breath.

There is a fourth kind of pranayama: this is the involuntary and natural cessation of breath.

When a man has reached a certain stage of spiritual development then his breathing in the midst of meditation may cease of its own accord at any time. This stoppage of breath may continue for many seconds or minutes. In the state of samadhi the breathing ceases altogether for hours at a time. There is no danger here, because it takes place only in man who has sufficiently developed spiritually and is able to sustain it. In any case he is seldom aware that breathing has ceased.

The final exercise recommended is the daily practice of watching the mind and how it works. The mind, being watched, finally becomes calmer. It becomes embarrassed as it were by its own silliness. This is mental control.

The object of pranayama is to arouse the kundalini. According to the philosophy of Raja Yoga the base of the spine has a huge reserve of spiritual or psychic energy, which is known also as the Serpent Power. It is known as the 'Coiled One' and thus it is also known as a serpent. When it is aroused the kundalini travels through the six psychic centers until it reaches the seventh center in the brain.

Ramakrishna explained the process thus:

> "The scriptures speak of seven centers of consciousness. When the mind is attached to worldliness it dwells in the three lower centers, at the navel, the organ of reproduction, and the organ of evacuation.
>
> "The fourth center is at the heart. When the mind dwells there man experiences his first spiritual awakening... Seeing this divine light he becomes filled with wonder and says, 'Ah, how blissful'.
>
> "The fifth center is at the throat. He whose mind has reached this center is freed from ignorance and delusion...
>
> "The sixth center is at the forehead. When the mind reaches this center there is direct vision of God... It is like a lantern; one feels as if one could touch the light, but cannot because of the pane of glass.
>
> "The seventh center is at the top of the head. When the mind reaches it samadhi is attained. One comes to know Brahman, united with Brahman."

Raja Yoga describes the human body as having only one life-force. And this power expresses itself in different ways at different levels of consciousness. These psychic areas are located in the *sushumna*, which is located in the center of the spinal column.

Vivkenanda described the awakening of the kundalini and its effects thus:

> "With the power of long internal meditation the vast mass of energy stored up travels along the sushumna

and strikes the center; the reaction is tremendous, immensely superior to the reaction of dream or imagination, immensely more intense that the reaction of sense perception... All worship, consciously or unconsciously, leads to this end. The man who thinks that he is receiving response to his prayers does not know that the fulfillment comes from his own nature, that he has succeeded by the mental attitude of prayer in waking up a bit of this infinite power which is coiled up within himself... "And yoga is the science of religion, the rationale of all worship, all prayers, forms, ceremonies and miracles."

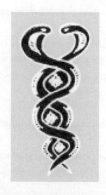

4

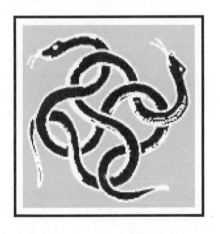

KRIYA YOGA : HISTORY

Kriya Yoga : History

Patanjali preserved yoga and its methods and techniques, but for a long time it was mostly practiced by spiritual aspirants privately and was taught secretly to disciples. The simple yoga involving pranayma became common but did not provide satisfactory results. Shivananda, the exponent of kundalini yoga, published books on kundalini, but it is so specialized and technical that few have taken it up.

And Kriya Yoga appears to have been forgotten, perhaps because of its secrecy and difficulty. There may have been a time when there was no proper disciple, to whom the secrets could be entrusted. There may have been a few, but who failed in getting initiated, and the secret system died with the gurus.

In 1861 Kriya Yoga was reintroduced by Babji, to the world through Lahiri Mahasaya, a householder and guru of the parents of Paramahansa Yogananda. Lahiri was initiated into the secret techniques of Kriya Yoga in the Himalaya. The encounter appears to be coincidental, but actually Babaji had been waiting for him there. It was not a chance encounter: Babaji had apparently known Lahiri in his previous life. And this time Lahiri was given the sacred assignment of spreading the philosophy and technique of Kriya Yoga.

"Bestow the Kriya Yoga only on qualified chelas (disciples)," Babaji instructed Lahiri. "He who vows to sacrifice all in the quest of the Divine is fit to unravel the final mysteries of life through the science of meditation."

Lahiri then asked his guru to relax the strict requirements and begged that it be given to sincere seekers, for there were many.

"Be it so. The divine wish has been expressed through you. Give kriya to all who humbly ask you for help," replied Babaji. But he required

Lahiri to give preparation period to those sincere seekers of the Absolute.

Kriya Yoga discipline is very strict. Today the Self-realization Fellowship in Los Angeles, California and the Yogoda Satsanga Society in India in Bihar require initiates to sign a pledge never to reveal the secrets of Kriya Yoga to others. It is to keep the system pure, in its original and uncorrupted form. Apparently Kriya Yoga has four stages of initiation. Disciples have to pass the first stage before being given the second stage initiation.

Kriya Yoga or any yoga method is for anyone who wishes to follow a spiritual path. It is not in conflict with any other creed, nor does it require extreme asceticism nor does it impose impossible difficulties. Traditional yoga was very difficult, but times have changed and yoga can be had or practiced by anyone who is sincere in his spiritual aspiration.

The term 'kriya' in its broad meaning is 'work' or 'method' or 'action' or even 'ritual'. And the broad meaning of 'Kriya Yoga' is 'Work towards Yoga.' There is just one science of yoga, the fundamental philosophy of which is 'Union with the Absolute', which means 'spiritual union', the ultimate goal of kriya.

There must have been just the original method, or ritual to attain yoga, but different 'kriyas' or methods or paths have evolved and developed as the different yogi masters struggled to find the most effective way. A plethora of methods sprang up besides the four major paths of yoga, which involved loving devotion, dedication to work and to God, intellectual analysis of what is Real, and the philosophical discourses on human life. There emerged on the spiritual landscape of India methods involving the psychophysical and physical disciplines which included Hatha Yoga, with its exercises which involved postures or mudras, pranayama and the chanting of mantras, and the use of the mandala in worship and in meditation.

This must be the natural evolution of the methods of yoga until all the essential work methods have been discovered. They vary and differ from each other but all with the same ultimate objective. With all these different methods the yogi masters must have inevitably tried one combination of techniques after another until they found what was suitable or the best for their disciples, or for the place and time. What was original in the form of worship, the ordinary and common remained, and this was not discarded. It was in the main the offering of sacrifices and therefore was ritualistic. The fire rituals, when perfectly worked out, proved effective in gaining their objectives in ritual worship. The rituals involving fire, and the invocations must have ended in a kind of meditative state, a mystical event, which brought a knowledge of the existence of the Absolute.

From these rituals yoga evolved and developed into a philosophy and a science. The form of worship was transformed as the objective was changed from beseeching for material security to spiritual security, the highest aim of worship, the ultimate as this does not merely secure life on earth but also life in the next world. It must have culminated in the mandala worship, which ultimately led into a deep meditative state. It retained the old ways and symbols. Worship involved the interaction of consciousness with the symbols in the mandala, which are encyclopedic, and hence, the necessity to be focused, for as the initiate moved in the mandala he had to concentrate on every step, on the thought that went into the act, in his movement.

In the end meditation alone remained the method to attain its goal, and for this reason yoga became both a philosophy and a science, the method which resulted in a mystical event, the union with the Absolute, which is known as self-realization, and which led to enlightenment. It is on this basis that it became known as a mystical science.

There are preliminary steps leading to meditation. The ordinary and most common are the practice of quieting the mind, the body and concentrating on breathing. There are other more involved techniques. Raja Yoga is regarded as one of the best, or the best of the medieval four major paths, because its practice involved a combination of more than a couple of preliminary techniques before meditation can be undertaken, but on the whole the flow from the preliminary steps into meditation proper is smooth: this makes up the whole process.

Any method in yoga is a science and sacred because its goal is spiritual. The Raja Yoga evolved mainly apparently also for highly evolved disciples, who needed a more advanced or highly specialized or technical system suitable for them. There are others with highly specialized techniques, exponents of which were yogi masters who have experimented with different combinations of disciplines. The original method as revealed in the Bhagavad Gita must have been called 'Kriya Yoga', but it must have developed into a highly specialized and technical method, and the name 'Kriya Yoga' , since it was the original was retained, and became a specific yoga method, which differed from other yoga systems. It is like any other scientific approach to

God-realization, but has developed a special technique, and thus offers a different approach to experience Reality. It is now claimed that with this specific kriya the goal can be achieved in a single lifetime.

All the yogic meditation systems in modern times are based on Patanjali's Yoga Sutras. Krishna earlier had introduced yoga and its techniques. In the middle of the 18th century Babaji, the mahavatar, introduced Kriya Yoga as a specific method to Lahiri Mahasaya, one of his more advanced disciples. He told him that the yoga science he was giving to the world was a revival of the same science that Krishna had given to Arjuna.

Krishna told Arjuna, his disciple and friend:

> " I proclaimed this imperishable yoga to ancient wise men, and makers of the law by which men are governed. They handed it down from one to another, through a line of royal sages, until this truth was lost to the world through a long lapse of time. The same ancient science I impart to you, for you are my disciple and friend, and this is the supreme secret."

This was apparently reintroduced to expedite the evolution of mankind and avoid the fate of the *Mahabaratta,* the great war in Bharat. Bharat was the ancient name of the subcontinent.

And this science was passed on to Lahiri's disciples, who included Sri Yukteswar, the guru of Paramahansa Yogananda. The latter introduced it in the United States. All yoga methods are based on Patanjali's sutras, but because different gurus developed their own methods their specific approach is traced to different guru-lines. The guru-line of Kriya Yoga is traced specifically to Babaji. It still practiced the ancient yoga tradition.

It has therefore remained pure, not mixed or modified with other methods. Babaji's yoga differs to a great extent from the ordinary and common, or other specialized methods. Basically its system is a combination of techniques, such as the use of mantra, concentration on sound and light, asanas or mudras, and kundalini exercises and pranayama.

The fundamental principles of Patanjali, basic in yoga, are followed, with would-be disciples chosen for their intelligence, character, and aptitude, and in the old yoga tradition they were tested for patience and perseverance for their dedication on the spiritual path. They were severely tested if they could be entrusted with the secrets of the discipline.

In today's yoga centers like the Self-Realization Fellowship in California the disciples, besides having the right credentials or qualification, are made to sign a pledge they will not reveal the Kriya Yoga method or processes to the uninitiated, or even to their classmates, for what instruction is given to each is personal and must be kept secret and not discussed freely.

Paramahansa Yogananda in his books refrained from revealing the secrets of Kriya Yoga, and so does some of his disciples who have written on the subject. They offer only a broad view of the system for the transmission of knowledge must be done orally by a guru. Thus this brief overview on the subject also gives only what has been culled from the reference materials. Some specialized techniques are given but not the entire procedure. It is perhaps only to show its technical aspects to exhibit its highly regarded system.

According to Sri Yukteswarji's book, *The Holy Science,* the world is moving away from Kali Yuga, the Dark Age, and is ascending the current electrical phase. For this reason people understand the philosophy and science of yoga, and experience within themselves the existence of fine elements and the subtle currents of prana. This is the reason why Kriya Yoga is suitable to this age.

INITIATION

In the old yoga tradition not everyone can be initiated into Kriya Yoga. They were examined for their intelligence, character and aptitude, and only those willing to renounce the world in their quest for enlightenment could be initiated. But Lahiri Mahasaya, a householder, interceded for his own disciples who were also householders, and who had their own family and social responsibilities to look after, and therefore who could not totally renounce or cut their link with the world.

Babaji relented and advised Lahiri to freely initiate all those who sincerely seek spiritual enlightenment. It was realized that householders and those with social responsibilities can inwardly be practicing renunciants; that is if they are not attracted and attached to things and actions and their effects.

Inner renunciation was regarded as more important than physical renunciation without inner transcendence. There was nevertheless the requirement for a preparatory period before they could be initiated.

Initiation means a new beginning. It is said that a person has passed through initiation when he experiences an awakening in consciousness, which results in greater understanding of life. In the old yoga tradition on the spiritual path the moment one experiences being born anew it is considered initiation.

True initiation is a spiritual baptism. This is the moment when a person fully commits himself to the rigorous discipline of yoga to experience the liberation of consciousness. The person who wants to follow the path of yoga must be willing to renounce thoughts, words, feelings and relationship, which are rooted in ego. And when one is finally accepted as a disciple and is initiated he is given instructions in philosophy, science, psychology and the conduct and procedure of meditation. The guru awakens his spirituality by means of *shaktipat*, the transmission of energy from guru to disciple, and the disciple is regarded as 'born' anew.

Once a disciple is initiated he must quit the old way of life and begin a new one, which is anchored in God. In the old tradition it took a long time for the guru to give the new disciple instructions in the scriptures, philosophy or the procedure in meditation. And very often the disciple wondered when he would finally be learning the secrets of yoga meditation. But he could not complain.

In fact the old guru was still testing him in body, mind and character. When the guru had satisfied himself that the disciple has the right patience and perseverance he to impart the secrets of yoga. This is mainly because the guru wants to be certain of his disciple's ability and capacity. He could not — was not allowed — to impart the secrets of yoga just to anyone.

In modern times this has changed. Today the disciple does not live with his guru like a son. Today he is on his own and out in the world. He is no longer being watched and observed by his guru. And today the secrets of yoga are freely given to him. He is no longer like a slave, serving his guru. But the initiate must be ready for a disciplined way of life to prepare himself for the experience of enlightenment. This is a basic requirement. He is a *vajragya,* a man of discrimination, out in the chaotic world which is more difficult than monastic life or living with the guru, for temptations abound. He is at the mercy of the world. Thus he has to prove that he is strong to the end till he attains his goal.

Those on the spiritual path of yoga are said not to be unduly affected by nature's influences. The kriya yogi returns consciousness to the Third Eye, and in this manner rises above external forces or circumstances. He can overcome all compulsive ties with the world.

GURU-DISCIPLE RELATIONSHIP

The guru-disciple relationship today is not a master-slave relationship as it used to be. The Sanskrit word 'guru' means 'that light which removes darkness'. The guru therefore is an enlightened man who can guide the disciple on the spiritual path to enlightenment.

In the old days for a young man to become a disciple was very difficult. Quite a few approached the guru, but very often only one was accepted: one whose intelligence, character and dedication had been tested. Hardship was extreme, but it was to test his patience, determination to continue, and his dedication and his faith in the guru. Only after a long time when the guru is certain of a disciple did he give him *diksha,* initiation, the first of four. In all these stages the disciple must prove his probity until the final stage when he passes the test.

In the yoga tradition the disciple, who has been chosen, and received initiation, surrenders everything to God and his guru, including his ego. He continues to live in his environment, but no longer as owner, but as a custodian or trustee. He is made to realize that everything belongs to God and he owns nothing. The surrendering of everything and receptiveness to the inner teachings and guidance of the guru was one of the tests of a disciple. Possession, selfishness and inability to surrender the ego to God and guru are great obstacles on the spiritual path. The path to self-realization or to heaven is indeed very difficult for people who cannot give up worldly possessions or their ego, and cannot abide by the rigorous discipline imposed on them as apprentices.

At times the guru-disciple relationship was carried to extremes. A guru can command a disciple to leap from a cliff down to the rocks below. It was to test his dedication and his faith in the guru. The disciple knows his guru will never put him in great danger. So he jumps. He dies on the rocks, but the guru brings him back to life. If a guru can do this he can also guide him to enlightenment and final liberation. In his determined and dedicated effort the disciple serves his guru in his apprenticeship sincerely and honestly with all his heart and mind, like a slave indeed. He gathers firewood, fetches water, cooks food, and does all the menial jobs for the guru, who in turn guides him and reveals the scriptures and the secrets of the way to final liberation.

Such a disciple will surely in time succeed his own guru and become a guru himself, enlightened. Thus the guru-line continues. The main role of a self-realized person is to be a light in the world, and to encourage others to awaken spiritually. Very often he becomes a guru. If no one can become a disciple according to the high standard set by the guru, the guru-line is terminated. The secrets of yoga cannot just be entrusted to anyone. Even if the guru-line ends with the last guru, it is better to have no successor guru than to have a false one who is really not enlightened.

But times have changed. The secret teachings, which were only meant for initiates are no longer kept secret. Anyone can be a disciple. Yoga meditation centers have proliferated with a plethora of diverging methods; they teach yogic meditation without the preliminary period required or the preliminary instructions required to undertake the science of meditation. In this modern age the secrets of the past are no longer secrets, but available without restrictions to anyone interested in learning and practicing yoga.

It offers the curious a chance to experiment and test the veracity and validity of the teachings. No one can do the checking or testing for him: he must do it alone. The books, or the guru, can only show him the way.

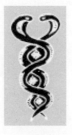

5

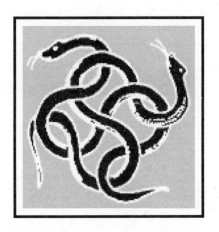

KRIYA YOGA : DISCIPLINE & TECHNIQUES

KRIYA YOGA : DISCIPLINE & TECHNIQUES

Kriya Yoga is a practical scientific method to purify the body, the thought-waves and the mind. The essential practice is concentration. And the process of achieving perfect concentration is by self-discipline, which involves control of the senses, analysis of the nature of consciousness, and the sense of surrendering to God self-consciousness, the sense of individuality or the ego-sense. This constitutes the path of Kriya Yoga.

Kriya Yoga applies the same rules and regulations on the development of virtue and restraints based on Patanjali's sutras. They are basic in all the different yoga methods and apply to all people. Observance of the law will not result in unfolding or transformation. Total surrender to the principles is what is required. This requirement entails purity of body, speech, thought and action, and worship of God must be done with the whole heart, mind and strength. Nothing is held back. God consumes the ego completely.

Love is also a fundamental requirement, as well as honesty and the intelligent use of available energies for higher purposes. Hence *brahmacharya* the conservation and right use of energies is also fundamental. This does not mean abstinence or celibacy. In Vedic times chelas or students led the life of brahmacharies but later married, and after fulfilling their social and familial obligations, returned to the practice of brahmacharya. This is actually the effort to attain self-mastery: this means neutralizing all passionate cravings of the sense, and not to be influenced by them.

The principle involved requires the intelligent use of vital energies, which are transmuted into finer essence called *ojas,* the agent that links the mental and the spiritual fields together. This is the principle that makes yogi's body develop a radiance and glow. A perfect body is not the goal of the discipline, but a positive by-product.

Physical and mental purity is the source of a serene and cheerful outlook in life. It makes the initiate able to control the senses and thus have the power of concentration. The Kriya Yoga technique of focusing on the Third Eye cleanses the mind of disturbing or unpleasant thoughts. The control of the mind gives him a choice how he will look at life and the world. He has this choice. No external power can control a person who has developed a mastery over his mind and body.

When self-realization is finally attained, supreme peace is enjoyed. When enlightenment dawns supreme happiness is experienced with abiding contentment at all times: there is perfect tranquility and even-mindedness. This experience of Reality brings in freedom.

As previously noted a disciple, after thorough examination and testing is finally given the first stage of initiation, and a disciple is regarded as newly born or 'born again', on the spiritual path. Spiritual education and training is now required. The old way of life is abandoned and a new one is adopted. His mother now is his guru who will teach and give him everything he needs. The guru is now his mother. The guru will pour into the newly-born all this teaching and he will not stop until he has succeeded in turning his 'son' into an enlightened man, a self-realized being.

The disciple is taught to be austere in his ways, given the scriptures to study, and to dedicate all the fruits of his labor to God. As in other yoga tradition Kriya Yoga teaches that the initiate must develop non-attachment to both painful and pleasant experiences. For no matter how pleasant an experience is it must be renounced, for it is transient, and when it disappears it leaves an unpleasant feeling, and the craving for it rises up once more. Ultimately it ends in pain. He is therefore taught that he must develop 'detachment' by simply remaining 'a witness of all that is observed' and by this method becomes uninvolved.

And when self-realization is finally attained even the sense of attachment to God must disappear. He is also taught to awaken to his own divine nature, and when he becomes self-aware, aware of his divine nature he unfolds in himself the power to be godlike. He must at all times be conscious of his divine nature: this is to keep himself centered in Being.

In addition to the cultivation of virtue, and the application of spiritual principles he is taught subjects such as cosmology — its emanation, preservation and dissolution – philosophy, psychology – including the study of the mind and consciousness – the study of the human body, including even the unseen psychic centers – and the presence of the divine in the heart. This study of kriya yoga is wide-ranging and incredibly vast. It seems incredible that one simple old guru could have such encyclopedic knowledge.

Kriya Yoga teaches that the real absolute force is the Mother Goddess who controls everything. It therefore also teaches science, not only of the macrocosm, but also the human body and its processes, the study of sound called mantra, the Sanskrit alphabet, and the planets and their movements, and their linkages revealing their integral unity as a whole and their influence on human life, and that everything has a governing principle. All these studies are concentrated on the mystery of human life. The ramifications of yoga is vast and its scope could cover the entire existential and experiential life of man.

The fundamental elements in the phenomenal universe are the three gunas: the sattva (stable), rajasa (dynamic) and tamasa (inert). All these elements have their gross, fine, subtle and primal nature. The spiritual path takes a man back to the primal nature, and hence the effect of intensive kriya yoga mediation makes the body of a yogi become refined until it becomes pure energy. There are therefore advanced yogis like Babaji who can dematerialize and materialize their body at will. The divine spark in the body is essentially pure, but to experience the phenomenal universe it must relate and link up through the mind with the physical body and the sense organs.

The doctrine of surrendering to God dissolves the ego and results in spiritual awakening. He must remain steadfast on the spiritual path, and at the same time must not be anxious for positive results. Like the karma yogi a spiritual aspirant must offer all the fruits of his work to God, and leave the rest to his will. The occasional perception or realization of truth about life is beneficial to the spiritual aspirant for this will lead eventually to the ultimate reality of worldly life, which begins to be seen merely as human drama, a 'dream-nature', just the play of light and shadow, with no power of its own to influence life, unless a man chooses to become emotionally involved.

In the Kriya Yoga system final enlightenment is attained in seven stages, which are apparently related to the seven chakras in the spinal column:

1. **First stage :** Awakening to knowledge one becomes conscious of obstacles that are to be removed on the spiritual path for unfoldment to be experienced. This awakening is actually an unfolding when he gains this insight. This is a positive sign.

2. **Second stage :** Awakening to knowledge the obstacles are neutralized by the aspirant's yogic effort. This is another positive sign. Knowledge has unfolded.

3. **Third Stage :** Samadhi is experienced. This is a further positive sign. Knowledge is unfolding progressively.

4. **Fourth stage :** During meditation knowledge is acquired and insight distinguishes the mind from the Self.

5. **Fifth stage :** With the awakened knowledge man can no longer be influenced by nature.

6. **Sixth stage :** When the yogi experiences transcending mind and body he becomes completely God-conscious. Nature's influence is dissolved, freedom is sensed.

7. **Seventh stage :** The yogi rests in the conscious experience of Pure Being — the unmanifest field of Pure Existence.

A free soul then lives in the world without being unduly influenced by it, or can transcend the realm of maya, and rest in the experience of being. He can remain God-conscious while watching the continuing drama around him without being caught up in it. Supremely enlightened souls are very free because they know that everything is a manifestation of consciousness, and therefore has no influence on him.

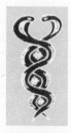

6

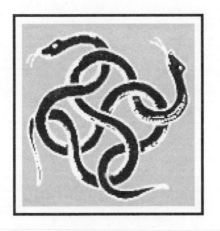

KRIYA YOGA
MEDITATION

KRIYA YOGA MEDITATION

Yoga meditation is a method of scientific experiment to verify and confirm the validity of the scriptural teachings. The aspirant takes on faith the guidance of his guru and proceeds to meditate to verify for himself the veracity and validity of the teachings of yoga.

Lahiri Mahasaya wrote:

> "Meditation on God is totally important to man's inner well-being. Meditation increases the flow of divine energy and grace within the entire nervous system and being. It clarifies the mental perspective, establishes emotional balance and inspires spiritual perceptions."

Five results in the practice of meditation:

First : Ignorance is removed by scriptural study and aspirant learns to discriminate. By discrimination the yogi detaches himself from earthly possessions and from his circle of friends. He severs all attachments because in the end he must forsake them. He now reclaims his divine birthright.

Second : He finds his consciousness and discovers he is imprisoned in the body and human consciousness.

Third : He now tries to silence the internal and external body sensations by detachment.

Fourth : He learns to make his breath quiet, also his heart, and focus his consciousness on the spine.

Fifth : He learns to withdraw attention from the heart, the muscles and the senses, and consciously put them to sleep. And joy is experienced.

KRIYA YOGA MEDITATION PROCEDURE

Sit comfortably in a quiet place, in a stable position in the padmasana posture with the feet drawn in and resting on the thighs; the body must be balanced with the head and neck erect and the spine straight.

It is advisable to sit on a woolen blanket for this enables a yogi to conserve energy during meditation. And he must face the east or north; it is apparently to take advantage of subtle magnetic currents which circulate around the planet. If the padmasana posture is difficult one can sit with the legs spread out but with the body balanced, the spine straight, and the head and neck erect. But generally even this to neophytes is very difficult. But a chair will do. The upright posture must be maintained. It is to allow the yogi to observe any kundalini activity in the lower spine.

This is followed by a quiet and calm moment, and God's presence is invoked. A simple short prayer is made for a successful meditation. For concentration he is advised to focus his eyes on the Third Eye, the point between the eyebrows, while he either begins pranayama or starts mantra-japa with a rosary.

The particular Kriya yoga method is to focus on the spiritual eye, the Third Eye, and in pranayama Kriya has introduced two syllable mantra: *hong - sau*. While focus is on the Third Eye the mantra is mentally uttered, in harmony with inhalation for the mantra *hong*, and exhalation for *sau*.

OM is the primary mantra. It is the primal sound that pervades the universe. It is the vibration and frequency of OM that is the origin of all sound in the cosmos, and therefore all other mantras. Mantra has become a science of sound. The OM mantra is the most powerful, but there are other mantras with the power to invite spiritual forces into the personal environment, and its main purpose is to invest on object of worship, such as a deity, with power; it is also to awaken latent forces in the human body.

Each chakra or psychic center has an individual energy frequency and its individual sound. In Kriya Yoga meditation the mantras are employed primarily to arouse the kundalini, the Serpent Power, coiled at the base of the spine. It is to make it rise up through the different chakras until it reaches the sahasrara chakra, the seventh psychic center at the crown of the head. But these mantras must be properly pronounced with their meanings known, otherwise the whole mantra will be ineffective.

Lahiri Mahasaya wrote on the Third Eye :

> "There is a sacred place within your body. It is the spiritual eye. It is the mystic door to God revelation. The light of God illuminates the entire consciousness. Within that effulgence is revealed a dark blue center. It is a vibrant light of solid blue. It is profoundly serene. Within the blue center shines a star, the guiding light of God. It is brilliant but soothing. It leads consciousness, the power of revelation and love into the glory of God-realization."

The kriya meditation process, even at the preliminary stage, is already complicated, for gaze is focused on the Third Eye, and in the pranayama process of inhalation the yogi must mentally utter 'hong' and in the outward breath he must mentally utter 'sau'. But as meditation progresses the body becomes increasingly relaxed, the vital energy becomes harmonized, and concentration becomes steady.

PRANAYAMA

Pranayama modifications or alterations are either external, internal or motionless. Breathing is mechanical and natural, but when the initiate begins to practice pranayama this natural and mechanical process is modified. External modification refers to the pause (stoppages of breath) after exhalation, and internal modification refers to the stoppage of breath after inhalation. Motionless modification refers to non-breathing by an act of will: it is stopping breathing consciously, but spontaneous breathlessness is also experienced during deep meditative state.

Modification of breath may be long or short. And this will effect the movement of prana, the luminous universal energy in breath, in the inner spaces of the body, then it is made to flow to the spine and the head. This is defined as cosmic breathing. This method expands awareness from the body-mind identification to cosmic consciousness.

The special kriya pranayama is known as yogic breathing, which is done through the sushumna, a tiny cavity in the center of the spinal chord. The process of breathing is through the nostrils, and feeling the air flow against the back of the throat, which is opened or expanded by rolling or dropping the tongue back. With the suction process of inward breathing the current of energy from the basal chakra can be made to ascend and flow to the spiritual eye. And when the air flows out through the nostrils the current descends back to the muladhara chakra. The spinal chord apparently becomes magnetized. The latent body energies are drawn to the spinal pathway and directed to the spiritual eye. This yogic breathing process can be of long or short duration. The experience is pleasant because prana is greater in amount than usual; it is revivifying.

Occasionally when the initiate is already advanced in the practice of kriya meditation technique and when prana is absorbed in the spiritual eye he may experience breathlessness, but there will still be a play of subtle prana throughout the body, maintaining it and ensuring its well-being.

Another technique in pranayama, special only to the kriya yoga method is the process of inhaling: this is also through the nostrils, with the breath made to pass through the medula oblongata at the base of the brain; this is to make it flow to the brain and then down the spinal chord; then this downward flow of energy current is reversed to flow back to the medula oblongata. This apparently will result in the perception of light at the spiritual eye. At the medula oblongata are five frequencies of vital energy reflected as light of the spiritual eye. They are also reflected in the body and regulated body processes. When they are drawn back to the spiritual eye they converge and form into a five-pointed star. Along with this light OM will be heard within.

The purpose is to clear the mind of mental modifications, thought-waves, which flow ceaselessly to make it incessantly busy. The meditation technique and continual practice weakens these thought-waves and they are said to become dormant, but perhaps really cleared away and the mind is described then as purified. The yogi then perceives the light: this is known as the Light of the Soul. It is also known as the Buddha Mind.

The light will appear, but the sound, when the yogi is focused on the light may not be heard unless concentration is focused on listening to it. In Kriya Yoga, when one has finally made some progress, the best spot to focus on is the crown chakra, the center of a thousand lotus petals. There will be a time when the initiate will experience transcendence – the Absolute Reality.

Another technique in pranayama is neutralizing inhalation and exhalation. This is another special method. It involves drawing up the energy current from the base chakra through the sushumna and letting it descend during exhalation. This neutralizes pranic flow and the yogi experiences calmness and even samadhi.

This procedure relaxes the body and the mind, the nervous system, decarbonizes the blood, with oxygen transmuted into pure energy and directed to flow to the chakras in the spine. The process will ultimately awaken the kundalini which is the primary purpose of pranayama.

When the kundalini is aroused the initiate will apparently hear the sound of OM. Kundalini has been described as serpent power because it resembles a coiled snake, and when aroused it hisses. It is the sibilant hissing sound that is heard.

In deep meditative state described as superconsciousness the initiate does not only enjoy peace and bliss but effects changes in the body on all levels. The body of a yogi is said to become radiant, the power of decay is neutralized, and he begins to radiate God into the environment.

The purpose of meditation is to transcend the world and overcome it. The phenomenal universe is really a play of light and shadow, a play or dream of God. It is thus said that life is only a dream. To experience liberation the initiate must die to the world and perceive that which is Unchanging. This is the ultimate goal.

When the mind has been purified the clear mental field itself must be transcended to experience the highest samadhi. And the truth is revealed. This experience is a 'revelation'. All that will remain is the conscious awareness of being in a blissful state. This takes time. For some it will take months perhaps, but on the whole it will take years, even decades, before this final ultimate experience of Reality can take place.

SAMADHI

Samadhi is said to take place when a yogi has attained yoga in deep meditative state. It is a condition when the initiate is no longer influenced by mental modifications, which are very disturbing. Actually it is a state when body sensations and mental thought-waves are absent and one is enveloped in an ineffable aura which is accompanied by a degree of awareness and a pleasant feeling. In this state the gunas or fundamental elements are in a state of equilibrium, and no longer unbalanced, and thus no longer active; they are said to be back in their original state of 'sat-chit-ananda' or 'consciousness-being-bliss'.

Attaining samadhi in deep meditation cleanses the mind, because superconsciousness results in enlightenment. Repeated practice of samadhi is the most purifying technique. This will establish firmly *sahaja samadhi*, a spontaneous awareness of truth at all times.

Samadhi is a state of intense awareness in which there is a degree of superconsciousness and one becomes increasingly self-realized: it is a state of supersensory awareness; it is not knowledge itself, but it enables a yogi to experience direct knowledge. Advanced yogis can leave their bodies at will by a special technique called , *mahasamadhi,* the great union or oneness. Because of this practice the fear of death disappears.

KRIYA YOGA PRECEPTS

The actual system of a human being, with six inner constellations revolving around the sun (the spiritual eye) is interrelated with the physical sun and the twelve constellations. All men are thus said to be affected by the inner and outer universes. This is the cosmic linkage.

In three years a Kriya yogi can accomplish by intelligent effort the same result that Nature brings to pass in one million years, the time that by nature a man requires to develop cosmic consciousness. With this kriya shortcut, however, a yogi must prepare his body and mind to withstand the power generated by intensive practice.

The average man's body is likened to a fifty-watt bulb, which cannot cope with the billion-watt power generated by the practice of Kriya. This practice of kriya meditation transforms a yogi's body until it is finally fit to accept the excessive power.

In man's natural life the flow of life energy is outward; the practice of kriya reverses the flow and guides it inward to strengthen the body and the brain cells. Man is not the body, but the soul. And Kriya Yoga is the scientific method to prove this: it is a system of spiritual enquiry.

Kriya Yoga is regarded as the real 'fire ritual'. This is the offering of sacrifice: it is figuratively in the fire sacrifice that the gross aspects of man are burned, and he is left lean in the eyes of mankind and of God. It reveals the full divinity of man; it is a holy sacred science, a way to discover the truth.

"Truth is not a theory, nor a speculative system of philosophy, nor an intellectual insight," wrote Paramahansa Yogananda. "Truth is in exact correspondence with reality. For man, truth is unshakable knowledge of his real nature, his Self or soul... It is to repossess or confirm his divine heritage."

Of the yogi the Bhagavad Gita says:

> "Steadfast a lamp burns sheltered from the wind;
> Such is the likeness of a yogi's mind –
> Shut from sense-storms and burning bright to Heaven,
> When mind broods placid, soothed with holy want;
> When self contemplates self, and in itself
> Hath comfort; when it knows the nameless joy
> Beyond all scope of sense, revealed to soul
> Only to soul! And, knowing, wavers not,
> True to the farther truth; when holding this,
> It deems no other treasure comparable,
> But, harbored there, cannot be stirred or shaken
> By any gravest grief, call that state 'peace',
> That happy severance yoga; call that man
> A perfect yogin."

Kriya Yoga Techniques

These yoga techniques have been culled from reference materials: they have apparently been given to emphasize the quality as a system of the Kriya Yoga discipline. However, the whole or complete technical processes are not given.

Mantra Meditation

A two-syllable mantra, the *hong-sau*, is usually given to a disciple. The disciple focussing on the spiritual eye listens mentally to the mantra *hong* when inhaling, and when exhaling to the mantra *sau*. Listening mentally to the mantra relaxes the mind, body and the nervous system, with the consequence of clearing the mental field. The mantra carries energy into deeper levels of the mind, and through the mantra alone full self-realization may be experienced.

Eventually as the disciple enters the threshold of the Silent Realm the mantra is forgotten: it drops away and he will find himself suddenly aware that a change has taken over his mind and body. At the beginning this may not be experienced; it may be sometime yet before the neophyte can experience anything.

After the mantra has dropped away the disciple may begin to see light in the spiritual eye and may even hear the sound of OM. Instruction in yogic meditation is for the disciple to focus on the light and sound at the same time and merge with either the light or the sound.

Inner Light & Sound Meditation

This appears to be the second stage of the kriya meditation. This takes place when the disciple enters the Silent Realm and the hong-sau mantra drops away. This is the moment when he begins to listen to the primary mantra OM, but at the initial stage he could only hear sounds, subtle one from the heart, and later from the chakras, but after sometime the mantra OM will eventually be heard.

Again for the neophyte this does not happen at the beginning: it will take time and a long practice in meditation, which will take days, or even weeks or months before he could hear the OM mantra. And it is not simply merging with it immediately for this is not possible. Merging with the sound will take some learning. And when success is achieved in merging with the sound it is dissolved, and this results to some degree in attaining cosmic-consciousness.

This to be transcended by merging with it until it is also dissolved, and samadhi is finally experienced.

It appears that meditation on light and sound is simultaneous: this is the impression one gets from the text. But this simply is not possible. One cannot immediately shift from light to sound: meditation on sound must be completed first, the whole sequence, until samadhi is attained.

INNER LIGHT MEDITATION

This is the third stage. Actually the beginner instructed to focus on the Third Eye while listening to the hong-sau mantra while simultaneously doing pranayama, will at first see no light even when the hong-sau mantra has dropped away, and he has entered the Silent Realm. It will take some time yet to see pieces of light. This is because the mental field has to be cleared of modifications. These pieces of light will eventually appear round with a black or blue dot in the center. It is small at first but this will eventually become larger.

When this appears one has to learn to merge with it until he attains again a degree of cosmic consciousness, which he has again to transcend to experience samadhi. The golden round light that looks like the sun is the Self that has to be realized. It will take years before it will appear suddenly and unexpectedly.

As has already been noted before taking up meditation the beginner is instructed on cleansing the mind of modifications for concentration. There are many requirements and rules and regulations to follow at each stage. It is not easy. Thus it requires patience and perseverance, but truly nothing is lost, only the steps taken will be followed by more until the ultimate goal has been achieved.

Kriya Yoga Pranayama

This is also known as kundalini pranayama or 'siddhi-pranayama'. The breathing processes are intended to arouse the kundalini coiled at the base of the spine, and when success follows psychic powers are said to be acquired; hence, the terms defining the system. 'Siddhi' means 'power'.

Breathing is the thread of life; it is the vital force that governs the entire body, its organs, the senses, the heart and the lungs, everything including the brain and mental activity or consciousness.

This pranayama system is also called 'yogic breathing'. It involves the modification or change in the normal auto-mechanical breathing. This breathing system is consciously controlled. The pause or stoppage of breathing after inhalation is called internal modification: this is actually called 'holding' and is to be longer than inhaling or exhaling. The pause after exhalation is called external modification. There is also the motionless modification when inhalation and exhalation are said to be neutralized.

Another technique is to roll the tongue back and make it drop down: this apparently enlarges the cavity in the back of the throat. One breathes through the nostrils and consciously makes the breath flow down the spinal chord through the sushumna, the tiny cavity in the spine. The pressure downward will force currents at the basal chakra rise up to the spiritual eye. On exhaling this current will drop down back to the base chakra.

This is the technique to awaken the kundalini, but it will take a long time before it could be aroused by this method. And because of this other methods, the application of mantras and the practice of asanas have been taken up as aids in awakening the Serpent Power.

The technique is initially taught apparently to make the prana flow up and down the spinal column and the spiritual eye. The result brings about the refinement of the nervous system and the brain, and in fact in the complete transformation of the body and the inner nature of man. This method assists and awakens the evolutionary process of man. In nature the purpose is for man to attain perfection, but by the natural process this will take hundreds of thousands of years. With this Kriya technique of pranayama there is a possibility that evolution of man toward perfection could be achieved in a single lifetime.

Shakti is the agent for this evolution in man; this is the feminine creative energy released when kundalini is awakened. Apparently as a result of a successful pranayama practice it can be made to circulate or directed by the inner intelligence. Hence, there is actually a great reservoir of creative evolutionary energy in the human body.

In Tantra the human body, the microcosm, is a complete replica of the phenomenal universe, the macrocosm. Everything in the universe is in the human body, including the possibility of evolving into a perfect being. This is what is being tapped by the ancient yogis: it is to bring about power and perfection.

ANOTHER ADVANCED TECHNIQUE

This involves a combination of pranayama, the use of mantra, and some head exercises or asanas. Shakti, the energy current, is brought up by pranayama to the heart chakra, around the heart, then the throat chakra, the spiritual eye, before to the crown chakra being brought up to.

Another is called the *kechari mudra:* the process is to direct the tip of the tongue behind the palate, then up to the head cavity. This results in profound superconsciousness. This is only for advanced yogis as it entails some danger. Some yogies in the old days made their final transition (this means quitting the body forever) by piercing the head cavity with the tip of their tongue.

REQUIREMENTS

Meditation is actually approaching God. Thus, the practice is to have a brief asanas in the morning and a bath before taking up meditation. God must be approached with a clean body and pure mind.

Practical Value

Meditation has also therapeutic effect upon the body and mind; it reduces stress, lowers high blood pressure, normalizes electrical patterns in the brain, relaxes the nervous system, and assists in the restoration of health and body function. People feel better, think more clearly and behave and conduct themselves normally, intelligently and peacefully.

It also shortens the period, which takes Nature to complete the evolution of man. Thus, with the practice of Kriya Yoga a man can fully develop into a perfect being in a few years instead of a hundred thousand years.

These higher and advanced techniques can be revealed only by the guru to their disciples, because they have already passed the lower and ordinary techniques and stages of meditation. The Samyama advanced techniques for advanced yogis are not given here, in particular the processes, which are anyway unknown except to the gurus. These advanced power-yoga processes could only be entrusted to pure disciples who could keep the secrets for themselves until there again crop up disciples to whom the secrets of the discipline could be passed on.

Note of Advice

Paramahansa Yogananda, one of the modern exponents of Kriya Yoga system, suggests that persons interested in following a spiritual path must stick to their particular religion, and limit themselves to just one method of yoga meditation.

It is a waste of energy and time when one tries one method after another. This is what he called 'spiritual window-shopping', which could end in confusion, dissatisfaction and loss of faith.

What is important is sincerity and faith in the spiritual quest. For even if the would-be disciple finds the best method but does not include faith and dedication the struggle would go nowhere.

The search must be conducted in his own heart for there Atman resides. And a guru, an enlightened master, can better guide him along the way on his personal lonely journey until his final destination is reached.

For more information on Kriya Yoga contact the following:

Self-Realization Fellowship
3880 San Rafael Avenue
Los Angeles
California 90065
USA

Yogada Satsanga Society
Paramahansa Yogananda Path
Ranchi 834001
Bihar, India

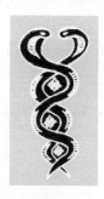

BIBLIOGRAPHY

Dasgupta, S.N, *Hindu Mysticism*, Motilal Banarsidas Publishers, Delhi, 1992.
*

Davis, Roy Eugene, *The Science of Kriya Yoga*, Tarapovevala, Bombay, 1984.

Metha, Dr Rohit, *The Science of Meditation*, Delhi, 1978.

Maury, Curt, *Folk Origins of Indian Art*, Columbia University Press, USA, 1969.

Prabhavananda, Swami, *Patanjali Yoga Sutras*, Ramakrishna Math, Madras, 1991.

Rao, S.N. Ramachandra, *Sri Chakra*, SW Satguru Publishers, Delhi, 1989.

Shivananda, *Kundalini*, India

Yogananda, Paramahansa, *Autobiography of a Yogi*, JAICO Publishing House, Delhi, 1974 reprint.

Other Titles in This Series by Book Faith India

1. SACRED SYMBOLS OF BUDDHISM — J.R. Santiago

2. SACRED SYMBOLS OF HINDUISM — J.R. Santiago

3. MANDALA: THE MYSTICAL DIAGRAM OF HINDUISM — J.R. Santiago

4. SACRED MANDALA OF BUDDHISM — J.R. Santiago

5. THANGKA: THE SACRED PAINTING OF TIBET — J.R. Santiago

For Catalog and more information Mail or Fax to:

PILGRIMS BOOK HOUSE
Mail Order, P.O.Box 3872, Kathmandu, Nepal
Fax: 977-1-424943
e-mail: mail@pilgrims.wlink.com.np
website: www.pilgrimsbooks.com